The Comprehensive Lean & Green Seafood And Veggie Cooking Guide

Healthy Seafood & Veggie Recipes For Beginners

Jesse Cohen

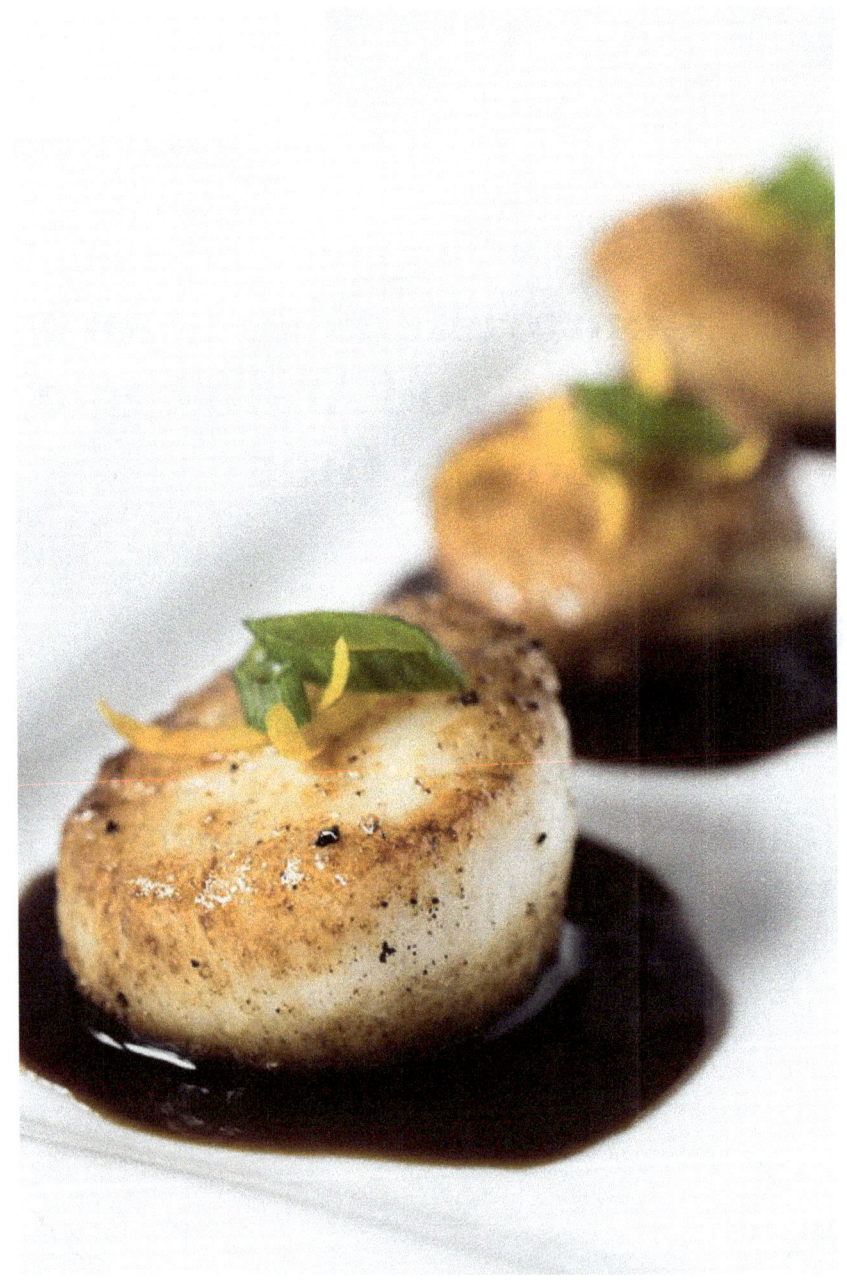

© **Copyright 2020 - All rights reserved.**

The content contained within this book may not be reproduced, duplicated or transmitted without direct written permission from the author or the publisher.

Under no circumstances will any blame or legal responsibility be held against the publisher, or author, for any damages, reparation, or monetary loss due to the information contained within this book. Either directly or indirectly.

Legal Notice:

This book is copyright protected. This book is only for personal use. You cannot amend, distribute, sell, use, quote or paraphrase any part, or the content within this book, without the consent of the author or publisher.

Disclaimer Notice:

Please note the information contained within this document is for educational and entertainment purposes only. All effort has been executed to present accurate, up to date, and reliable, complete information. No warranties of any kind are declared or implied. Readers acknowledge that the author is not engaging in the rendering of legal, financial, medical or professional advice. The content within this book has been derived from various sources. Please consult a licensed professional before attempting any techniques outlined in this book.

By reading this document, the reader agrees that under no circumstances is the author responsible for any losses, direct or indirect, which are incurred as a result of the use of information contained within this document, including, but not limited to, — errors, omissions, or inaccuracies.

Table of contents

Zesty Salmon 7

Stuffed Salmon 9

Salmon with Asparagus 12

Salmon Parcel 14

Salmon with Cauliflower Mash 16

Salmon with Salsa 18

Walnut Crusted Salmon 20

Garlicky Tilapia 22

Tilapia Piccata 23

Cod in Dill Sauce 25

Cod & Veggies Bake 27

Cod & Veggie Pizza 29

Garlicky Haddock 32

Haddock in Parsley Sauce 34

Halibut with Zucchini 35

Roasted Mackerel 37

Herbed Sea Bass 39

Lemony Trout 41

Tuna Stuffed Avocado 43

Fish & Spinach Curry 44

Crab Cakes 46

Shrimp Lettuce Wraps 48

Shrimp Kabobs	49
Shrimp with Zucchini Noodles	51
Shrimp with Spinach	53
Shrimp with Broccoli & Carrot	55
Shrimp, Spinach & Tomato Casserole	57
Prawns with Bell Pepper	59
Prawns with Broccoli	61
Prawns with Asparagus	63
Prawns with Kale	65
Scallops with Broccoli	67
Scallops with Asparagus	69
Scallops with Spinach	71
Shrimp & Scallops with Veggies	73
Vegetarian Burgers	75
Cauliflower with Peas	77
Broccoli with Bell Peppers	79
Veggies Curry	80
Veggies Combo	82
Cauliflower with Peas	84
Bok Choy & Mushroom Stir Fry	86
Broccoli with Bell Peppers	88
Stuffed Zucchini	90
Zucchini & Bell Pepper Curry	92
Zucchini Noodles with Mushroom Sauce	94

Squash Casserole 96

Veggies & Walnut Loaf 98

Tofu & Veggie Burgers 101

Tofu & Veggie Lettuce Wraps 104

Tofu with Kale 106

Zesty Salmon

Servings: 4

Preparation Time: 10 minutes

Cooking Time: 10 minutes

Ingredients:

- 1 tablespoon of butter, melted
- 1 tablespoon of fresh lemon juice
- 1 teaspoon of Worcestershire sauce
- 1 teaspoon of lemon zest, grated finely
- 4 (6-ounce of) salmon fillets
- Salt and ground black pepper, to taste

Instructions:

1. In a baking dish, place butter, juice, Worcester sauce, and lemon peel, and blend well.
2. Coat the fillets with the mixture then arrange skin side-up in the baking dish.
3. Put aside for about 15 minutes.
4. Preheat the broiler of oven.
5. Arrange the oven rack about 6-inch from the element.
6. Line a broiler pan with a bit of foil.

7. Remove the salmon fillets from baking dish and season with salt and black pepper.
8. Arrange the salmon fillets onto the prepared broiler pan, skin side down.
9. Broil for about 8-10 minutes.
10. Serve hot.

Stuffed Salmon

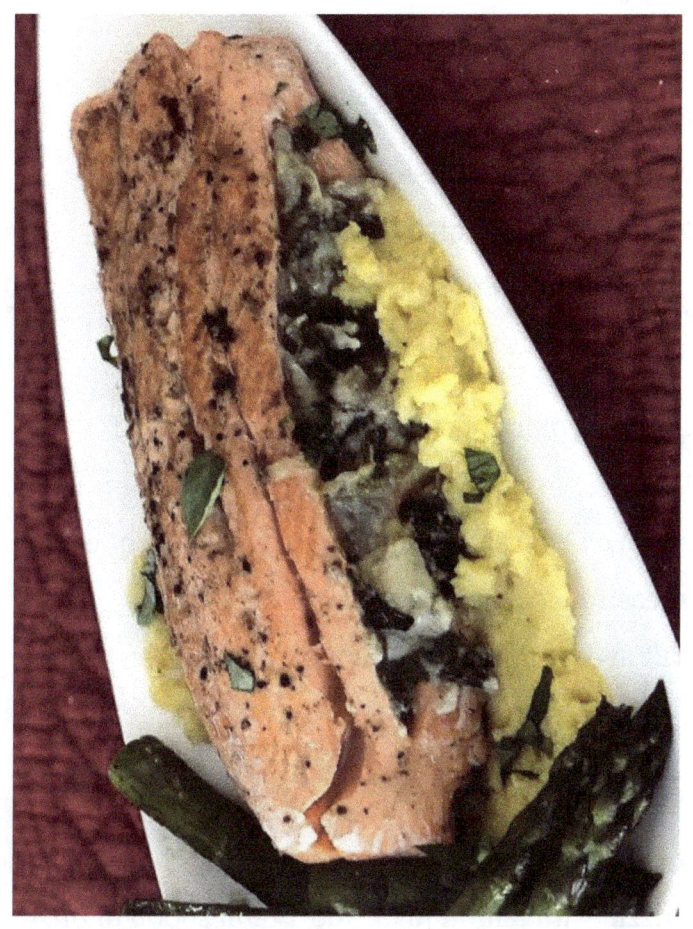

Servings: 4

Preparation Time: 15 minutes

Cooking Time: 16 minutes

Ingredients:

For Salmon:

- 4 (6-ounce of) skinless salmon fillets
- Salt and ground black pepper, as required
- 2 tablespoons of fresh lemon juice
- 2 tablespoons of olive oil, divided
- 1 tablespoon of unsalted butter

For Filling:

- 4 ounces of low-fat cream cheese, softened
- ¼ cup of low-fat Parmesan cheese, grated finely
- 4 ounces of frozen spinach, thawed and squeezed
- 2 teaspoons of garlic, minced
- Salt and ground black pepper, as required

Instructions:

1. Season each salmon fillet with salt and black pepper then, drizzle with lemon juice and 1 tablespoon of oil.
2. Arrange the salmon fillets onto a smooth surface.
3. With a pointy knife, cut a pocket into each salmon fillet about ¾ of the way through, being careful not to cut all the way.

4. For filling: In a bowl, add the cream cheese, Parmesan cheese, spinach, garlic, salt and black pepper and blend well.
5. Place about 1-2 tablespoons of spinach mixture into each salmon pocket and spread evenly.
6. In a skillet, heat the remaining oil and butter over medium-high heat and cook the salmon fillets for about 6-8 minutes per side.
7. Remove the salmon fillets from heat and transfer onto the serving plates.
8. Serve immediately.

Salmon with Asparagus

Servings: 6

Preparation Time: 10 minutes

Cooking Time: 20 minutes

Ingredients:

- 6 (4-ounce of) salmon fillets
- 2 tablespoons of extra-virgin olive oil
- 3 tablespoons of fresh parsley, minced
- ¼ teaspoon of ginger powder
- Salt and freshly ground black pepper, to taste
- 1½ pounds fresh asparagus

Instructions:

1. Preheat your oven to 400 degrees.
2. Grease a large baking dish.
3. In a bowl, place all ingredients and blend well.
4. Arrange the salmon fillets into the prepared baking dish in a single layer.
5. Bake for about 15-20 minutes or until the desired doneness of salmon.

6. Meanwhile, in a pan of the boiling water, add asparagus and cook for about 4-5 minutes.
7. Drain the asparagus well.
8. Divide the asparagus onto serving plates evenly and top each with 1 salmon fillet and serve.

Salmon Parcel

Servings: 6

Preparation Time: 15 minutes

Cooking Time: 20 minutes

Ingredients:

- 6 (4-ounce of) salmon fillets
- Salt and freshly ground black pepper, to taste
- 1 yellow bell pepper, seeded and cubed
- 1 red bell pepper, seeded and cubed
- 4 plum tomatoes, cubed
- 1 small onion, sliced thinly
- ½ cup of fresh parsley, chopped
- ¼ cup of extra-virgin olive oil
- 2 tablespoons of fresh lemon juice

Instructions:

1. Preheat your oven to 400 degrees F.
2. Arrange 6 pieces of foil onto a smooth surface.
3. Place 1 salmon fillet on each bit of foil and sprinkle with salt and black pepper.
4. In a bowl, mix bell peppers, tomato and onion.

5. Place veggie mixture over each fillet evenly and top with parsley and capers evenly.
6. Drizzle with oil and lemon juice.
7. Fold each bit of foil around the salmon mixture to seal it.
8. Arrange the foil packets onto a large baking sheet in a single layer.
9. Bake for about 25 minutes.
10. Remove from the oven and place the foil packets onto serving plates.
11. Carefully unwrap each foil packet and serve.

Salmon with Cauliflower Mash

Servings: 4

Preparation Time: 15 minutes

Cooking Time: 20 minutes

Ingredients:

For Cauliflower Mash:

- 1-pound cauliflower, cut into florets
- 1 tablespoon of extra-virgin olive oil
- 3 garlic cloves, minced
- 1 teaspoon of fresh thyme leaves
- Salt and freshly ground black pepper, to taste

For Salmon:

- 1 (1-inch) piece fresh ginger, grated finely
- 1 tablespoon of honey
- 1 tablespoon of fresh lemon juice
- 1 tablespoon of Dijon mustard
- 2 tablespoons of olive oil
- 4 (6-ounce of) salmon fillets
- 2 tablespoons of fresh parsley, chopped

Instructions:

1. For mash: In a large saucepan of water, arrange a steamer basket and bring to a boil.
2. Place the cauliflower florets in a steamer basket and steam covered for about 10 minutes.
3. Drain the cauliflower and put aside.
4. In a small frying pan, heat the oil over medium heat and sauté the garlic for about 2 minutes.
5. Remove the frying pan from heat and transfer the garlic oil in a large food processor.
6. Add the cauliflower, thyme, salt and black pepper and pulse until smooth.
7. Transfer the cauliflower mash into a bowl and put aside.
8. Meanwhile, in a bowl, mix ginger, honey, juice and Dijon mustard. Set aside.
9. In a large non-stick skillet, heat vegetable oil over medium-high heat and cook the salmon fillets for about 3-4 minutes per side.
10. Stir in honey mixture and immediately remove from heat.
11. Divide warm cauliflower mash onto serving plates.
12. Top each plate with 1 salmon fillet and serve.

Salmon with Salsa

Servings: 4

Preparation Time: 15 minutes

Cooking Time: 8 minutes

Ingredients:

For Salsa:

- 2 large ripe avocados, peeled, pitted and cut into small chunks
- 1 small tomato, chopped
- 2 tablespoons of red onion, chopped finely
- ¼ cup of fresh cilantro, chopped finely
- 1 tablespoon of jalapeño pepper, seeded and minced finely
- 1 garlic clove, minced finely
- 3 tablespoon of fresh lime juice
- Salt and ground black pepper, as required

For Salmon:

- 4 (5-ounce of) (1-inch thick) salmon fillets
- Sea salt and ground black pepper, as required
- 3 tablespoons of olive oil
- 1 tablespoon of fresh rosemary leaves, chopped

- 1 tablespoon of fresh lemon juice

Instructions:

1. For salsa: add all ingredients in a bowl and gently, stir to mix.
2. With a plastic wrap, cover the bowl and refrigerate before serving.
3. For salmon: season each salmon fillet with salt and black pepper generously.
4. In a large skillet, heat the oil over medium-high heat.
5. Place the salmon fillets, skins side up and cook for about 4 minutes.
6. Carefully change the side of every salmon fillet and cook for about 4 minutes more.
7. Stir in the rosemary and juice and take away from the heat.
8. Divide the salsa onto serving plates evenly.
9. to every plate with 1 salmon fillet and serve.

Walnut Crusted Salmon

Servings: 2

Preparation Time: 15 minutes

Cooking Time: 20 minutes

Ingredients:

- ½ cup of walnuts
- 1 tablespoon of fresh dill, chopped
- 2 tablespoons of fresh lemon rind, grated
- Salt and ground black pepper, as required
- 1 tablespoon of coconut oil, melted
- 3-4 tablespoons of Dijon mustard
- 4 (3-ounce of) salmon fillets
- 4 teaspoons of fresh lemon juice
- 3 cups of fresh baby spinach

Instructions:

1. Preheat your oven to 350 degrees F.
2. Line a large baking sheet with parchment paper.
3. Place the walnuts in a food processor and pulse until chopped roughly.

4. Add the dill, lemon peel, garlic salt, black pepper, butter, and pulse until a crumbly mixture forms.
5. Place the salmon fillets onto the prepared baking sheet in a single layer, skin-side down.
6. Coat the top of every salmon fillet with Dijon mustard.
7. Place the walnut mixture over each fillet and gently, press into the surface of salmon.
8. Bake for about 15–20 minutes.
9. Remove the salmon fillets from the oven and transfer onto the serving plates.
10. Drizzle with the juice and serve alongside the spinach.

Garlicky Tilapia

Servings: 4

Preparation Time: 10 minutes

Cooking Time: 5 minutes

Ingredients:

- 2 tablespoons of olive oil
- 4 (5-ounce of) tilapia fillets
- 3 garlic cloves, minced
- 1 tablespoon of fresh ginger, minced
- 2-3 tablespoons of low-sodium chicken broth
- Salt and ground black pepper, to taste
- 6 cups of fresh baby spinach

Instructions:

1. In a large sauté pan, heat the oil over medium heat and cook the tilapia fillets for about 3 minutes.
2. Flip the side and stir in the garlic and ginger.
3. Cook for about 1-2 minutes.
4. Add the broth and cook for about 2-3 more minutes.
5. Stir in salt and black pepper and take away from heat.
6. Serve hot alongside the spinach.

Tilapia Piccata

Servings: 4

Preparation Time: 15 minutes

Cooking Time: 8 minutes

Ingredients:

- 3 tablespoons of fresh lemon juice
- 2 tablespoons of olive oil
- 2 garlic cloves, minced
- ½ teaspoon of lemon zest, grated
- 2 teaspoons of capers, drained
- 2 tablespoons of fresh basil, minced
- 4 (6-ounce of) tilapia fillets
- Salt and ground black pepper, as required
- 6 cups of fresh baby kale

Instructions:

1. Preheat the broiler of the oven.
2. Arrange an oven rack about 4-inch from the heating element.
3. Grease a broiler pan.

4. In a small bowl, add the lemon juice, oil, garlic and lemon peel and beat until well combined.
5. Add the capers and basil and stir to mix.
6. Reserve 2 tablespoons of mixture in a small bowl.
7. Coat the fish fillets with remaining capers mixture and sprinkle with salt and black pepper.
8. Place the tilapia fillets onto the broiler pan and broil for about 3-4 minutes side.
9. Remove from the oven and place the fish fillets onto serving plates.
10. Drizzle with reserved capers mixture and serve alongside the kale.

Cod in Dill Sauce

Servings: 2

Preparation Time: 10 minutes

Cooking Time: 13 minutes

Ingredients:

- 2 (6-ounce of) cod fillets
- 1 teaspoon of onion powder
- Salt and ground black pepper, as required
- 3 tablespoons of butter, divided
- 2 garlic cloves, minced
- 1-2 lemon slices
- 2 teaspoons of fresh dill weed
- 3 cups of fresh spinach, torn

Instructions:

1. Season each cod fillet evenly with the onion powder, salt and black pepper.
2. In a medium skillet, heat 1 tablespoon of oil over high heat and cook the cod fillets for about 4-5 minutes per side.
3. Transfer the cod fillets onto a plate.

4. Meanwhile, in a frying pan, heat the remaining oil over low heat and sauté the garlic and lemon slices for about 40-60 seconds.
5. Stir in the cooked cod fillets and dill and cook, covered for about 1-2 minutes.
6. Remove the cod fillets from heat and transfer onto the serving plates.
7. Top with the pan sauce and serve immediately alongside the spinach.

Cod & Veggies Bake

Servings: 4

Preparation Time: 15 minutes

Cooking Time: 20 minutes

Ingredients:

- 1 teaspoon of olive oil
- ½ cup of onion, minced
- 1 cup of zucchini, chopped
- 1 garlic clove, minced
- 2 tablespoons of fresh basil, chopped
- 2 cups of fresh tomatoes, chopped
- Salt and ground black pepper, as required
- 4 (6-ounce of) cod steaks
- 1/3 cup of feta cheese, crumbled

Instructions:

1. Preheat your oven to 450 degrees F.
2. Grease a large shallow baking dish.
3. In a skillet, heat oil over medium heat and sauté the onion, zucchini and garlic for about 4-5 minutes.

4. Stir in the basil, tomatoes, salt and black pepper and immediately remove from heat.
5. Place the cod steaks into the prepared baking dish in a single layer and top with tomato mixture evenly.
6. Sprinkle with the cheese evenly.
7. Bake for about 15 minutes or until desired doneness.
8. Serve hot.

Cod & Veggie Pizza

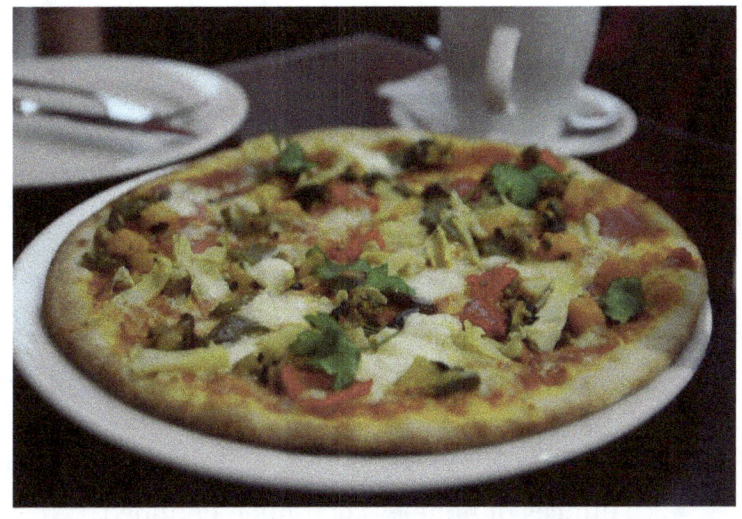

Servings: 3

Preparation Time: 20 minutes

Cooking Time: 1 hour

Ingredients:

For Base:

- Olive oil cooking spray
- ¼ cup of oat flour
- 2 teaspoons of dried rosemary, crushed
- Freshly ground black pepper, to taste
- 4 egg whites

- 2½ teaspoons of olive oil
- ½ cup of low-fat Parmesan cheese, grated freshly
- 2 cups of zucchini, grated and squeezed

For Topping:

- 1 cup of tomato paste
- 1 teaspoon of fresh rosemary, minced
- 1 teaspoon of fresh basil, minced
- Freshly ground black pepper, to taste
- 4 cups of fresh mushrooms, chopped
- 1 tomato, chopped
- 3 ounces of boneless cod fillet, chopped
- 1½ cups of onion, sliced into rings
- 1 red bell pepper, seeded and chopped
- 1 green bell pepper, seeded and chopped
- 1/3 cup of low-fat mozzarella, shredded

Instructions:

1. Preheat your oven to 400 degrees F.
2. Grease a pie dish with cooking spray.
3. For base: in a large bowl, add all the ingredients and blend until well combined.
4. Transfer the mixture into the prepared pie dish and press to smooth the surface.

5. Bake for about 40 minutes.
6. Remove from the oven and put aside to chill for at least 15 minutes.
7. Carefully end up the crust onto a baking sheet.
8. For topping: in a bowl, add tomato paste, herbs and black pepper.
9. Spread spaghetti sauce mixture over the crust evenly.
10. Arrange the vegetables over spaghetti sauce, followed by the cheese.
11. Bake for about 20 minutes or until cheese is melted.
12. Serve hot.

Garlicky Haddock

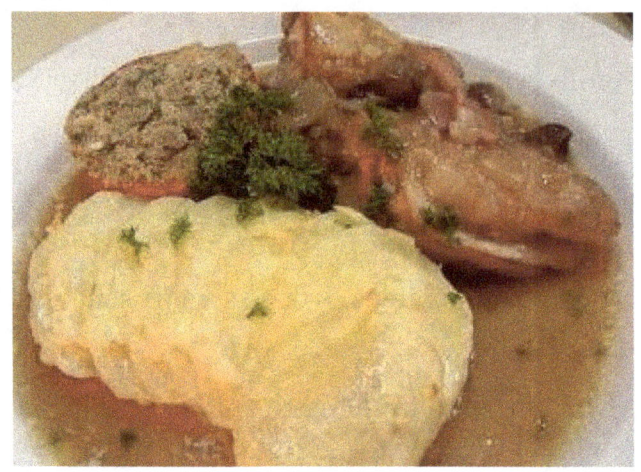

Servings: 2

Preparation Time: 10 minutes

Cooking Time: 11 minutes

Ingredients:

- 2 tablespoons of olive oil, divided
- 4 garlic cloves, minced and divided
- 1 teaspoon of fresh ginger, grated finely
- 2 (4-ounce of) haddock fillets
- Salt and freshly ground black pepper, to taste
- 3 cup of fresh baby spinach

Instructions:

1. In a skillet, heat 1 tablespoon of oil over medium heat and sauté 2 garlic cloves and ginger for about 1 minute.
2. Add the haddock fillets, salt and black pepper and cook for about 3-5 minutes per side or until desired doneness.
3. Meanwhile, in another skillet, heat remaining oil over medium heat and heat and sauté remaining garlic for about 1 minute.
4. Add the spinach, salt and black pepper and cook for about 4-5 minutes.
5. Divide the spinach onto serving plates and top each with 1 haddock fillet.
6. Serve immediately.

Haddock in Parsley Sauce

Servings: 2

Preparation Time: 10 minutes

Cooking Time: 9 minutes

Ingredients:

- 2 (5-ounce of) haddock fillets
- Salt and ground black pepper, as required
- 2 tablespoons of olive oil
- 1 tablespoon of fresh parsley, chopped
- 1 tablespoon of fresh lime juice
- 3 cups of fresh arugula

Instructions:

1. In a large skillet, heat the oil over medium-high heat.
2. Place the haddock fillets, skins side up and cook for about 4 minutes.
3. Carefully change the side of every fillet and cook for about 4 minutes more.
4. Stir in the parsley and juice and take away from the heat.
5. Serve hot alongside the arugula.

Halibut with Zucchini

Servings: 4

Preparation Time: 15 minutes

Cooking Time: 20 minutes

Ingredients:

- 1 teaspoon of olive oil
- ½ cup of yellow onion, minced
- 1 cup of zucchini, chopped
- 2 garlic cloves, minced
- 2 tablespoons of fresh basil, chopped
- 2 cups of fresh tomatoes, chopped
- Salt and freshly ground black pepper, to taste
- 4 (6-ounce) of halibut steaks
- 1/3 cup of feta cheese, crumbled

Instructions:

1. Preheat your oven to 450 degrees F.
2. Grease a large shallow baking dish.
3. In a skillet, heat the oil over medium heat and sauté the onion, zucchini and garlic for about 4-5 minutes.

4. Stir in the basil, tomatoes and black pepper and immediately remove from heat.
5. Place the halibut steaks into the prepared baking dish in a single layer.
6. Top with the tomato mixture evenly and sprinkle with cheese evenly.
7. Bake for about 15 minutes or until desired doneness.
8. Serve hot.

Roasted Mackerel

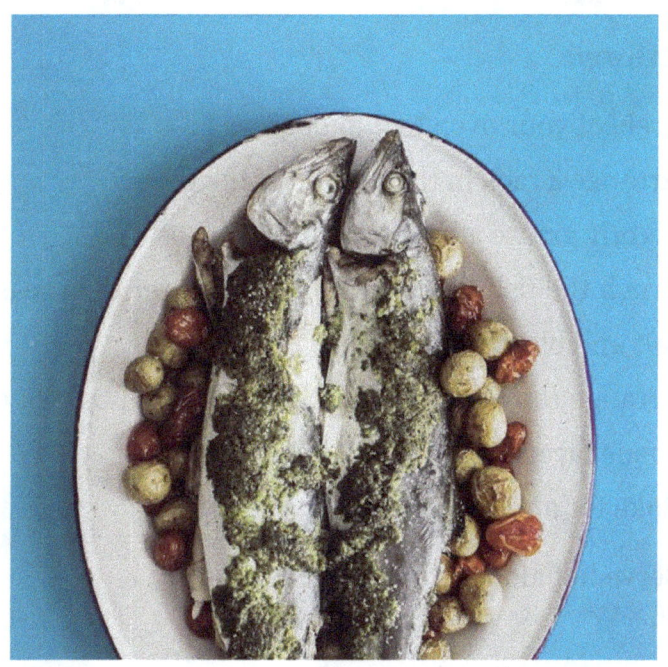

Servings: 2

Preparation Time: 10 minutes

Cooking Time: 20 minutes

Ingredients:

- 2 (7-ounce of) mackerel fillets
- 1 tablespoon of olive oil
- Salt and ground black pepper, to taste

- 3 cups of fresh baby greens

Instructions:

1. Preheat your oven to 350 degrees F.
2. Arrange a rack in the middle of the oven.
3. Lightly grease a baking dish.
4. Brush the fish fillets with melted butter then season with salt and black pepper.
5. Arrange the fish fillets into the prepared baking dish in a single layer.
6. Bake for about 20 minutes.
7. Serve hot alongside the greens.

Herbed Sea Bass

Servings: 2

Preparation Time: 10 minutes

Cooking Time: 20 minutes

Ingredients:

- 2 (1¼-pound) whole sea bass, gutted, gilled, scaled and fins removed
- Salt and ground black pepper, as required
- 6 fresh bay leaves
- 2 fresh thyme sprigs
- 2 fresh parsley sprigs
- 2 fresh rosemary sprigs
- 2 tablespoons of butter, melted
- 2 tablespoons of fresh lemon juice
- 3 cups of fresh arugula

Instructions:

1. Season the cavity and outer side of every fish with salt and black pepper evenly.
2. With a plastic wrap, cover each fish and refrigerate for 1 hour.

3. Preheat the oven to 450 degrees F.
4. Lightly grease a baking dish.
5. Arrange 2 bay leaves in the bottom of the prepared baking dish.
6. Divide herb sprigs and remaining bay leaves inside the cavity of every fish.
7. Arrange both fish over bay leave in the baking dish and drizzle with butter.
8. Roast for about 15-20 minutes or until fish is cooked through.
9. Remove the baking dish from oven and place the fish onto a platter.
10. Drizzle the fish with juice and serve alongside the arugula.

Lemony Trout

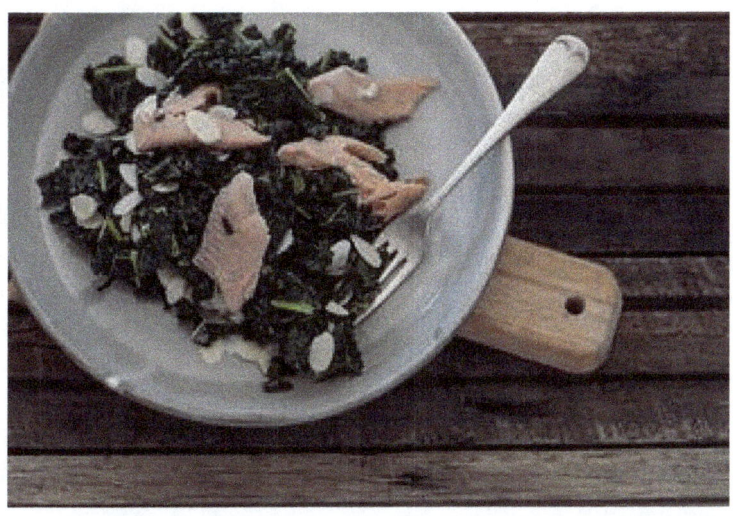

Servings: 4

Preparation Time: 15 minutes

Cooking Time: 25 minutes

Ingredients:

- 2 (1½-pound) wild-caught trout, gutted and cleaned
- Salt and ground black pepper, as required
- 1 lemon, sliced
- 2 tablespoons of fresh dill, minced
- 2 tablespoon of butter, melted
- 2 tablespoons of fresh lemon juice

Instructions:

1. Preheat the oven to 475 degrees F.
2. Arrange a wire rack onto a foil-lined baking sheet.
3. Sprinkle the trout with salt and black pepper from inside and out of doors generously.
4. Fill the cavity of every fish with lemon slices and dill.
5. Place the trout onto the prepared baking sheet and drizzle with the melted butter and lemon juice.
6. Bake for about 25 minutes.
7. Remove the baking sheet from oven and transfer the trout onto a serving platter.
8. Serve hot.

Tuna Stuffed Avocado

Servings: 2

Preparation Time: 15 minutes

Ingredients:

- 1 large avocado, halved and pitted
- 1 tablespoon of onion, chopped finely
- 2 tablespoons of fresh lemon juice
- 5 ounces of cooked tuna, chopped
- Salt and ground black pepper, as required

Instructions:

1. With a spoon, scoop out the flesh from the centre of every avocado half and transfer into a bowl.
2. Add the onion and juice and mash until well combined.
3. Add tuna, salt and black pepper and stir to mix.
4. Divide the tuna mixture into both avocado halves evenly and serve immediately.

Fish & Spinach Curry

Servings: 4

Preparation Time: 15 minutes

Cooking Time: 15 minutes

Ingredients:

- 1 tablespoon of coconut oil
- 1 small yellow onion, chopped
- 2 garlic cloves, minced
- 1 teaspoon of fresh ginger, minced
- 1 large tomato, peeled and chopped
- 1 tablespoon of curry powder
- ¼ cup of water
- 1¼ cups of unsweetened coconut milk
- 1-pound of skinless grouper fillets, cubed into 2-inch size
- ¾ pound of fresh spinach, chopped
- Salt, as required
- 2 tablespoons of fresh parsley, chopped

Instructions:

1. In a large wok, melt the coconut oil over medium heat and sauté the onion, garlic and ginger for about 5 minutes.

2. Add the tomatoes and curry powder and cook for about 2-3 minutes, crushing with the rear of the spoon.
3. Add the water and coconut milk and bring to a mild boil.
4. Stir in grouper pieces and spinach and cook for about 4-5 minutes.
5. Stir in the salt and parsley and serve hot.

Crab Cakes

Servings: 4

Preparation Time: 15 minutes

Cooking Time: 28 minutes

Ingredients:

For Crab Cakes:

- 2 tablespoons of olive oil, divided
- ½ cup of onion, chopped finely
- 3 tablespoons of blanched almond flour
- ¼ cup of egg whites
- 2 tablespoons of mayonnaise
- 1 tablespoon of dried parsley, crushed
- 1 teaspoon of yellow mustard
- 1 teaspoon of Worcestershire sauce
- 1 tablespoon of Old Bay seasoning
- Salt and ground black pepper, to taste
- 1-pound lump crabmeat, drained

For Salad:

- 5 cups of fresh baby arugula
- 2 tomatoes, chopped

- 2 tablespoons of olive oil
- Salt and ground black pepper, to taste

Instructions:

1. For crab cakes: Heat 2 teaspoons of olive oil in a wok over medium heat and sauté onion for about 8-10 minutes.
2. Remove the frying pan from heat and put aside to chill slightly.
3. Place cooked onion and remaining ingredients apart from crabmeat in a bowl and blend until well combined.
4. Add the crabmeat and gently, stir to mix.
5. Make 8 equal-sized patties from the mixture.
6. Arrange the patties onto a foil-lined tray and refrigerate for about 30 minutes.
7. In a large frying pan, heat remaining oil over medium-low heat and cook patties in 2 batches for about 3-4 minutes per side or until desired doneness.
8. For Salad: In a bowl, add all ingredients, and toss to coat well.
9. Divide salad onto serving plates and to every with 2 patties.
10. Serve immediately.

Shrimp Lettuce Wraps

Servings: 4

Preparation Time: 15 minutes

Cooking Time: 25 minutes

Ingredients:

- 1 teaspoon of extra-virgin olive oil
- 1 garlic clove, minced
- 1½ pounds shrimp, peeled, deveined and chopped
- Salt, as required
- 8 large lettuce leaves
- 1 tablespoon of fresh chives, minced

Instructions:

1. In a large sauté pan, heat the vegetable oil over medium heat and sauté garlic for about 1 minute.
2. Add the shrimp and cook for about 3-4 minutes.
3. Remove from heat and put aside to chill slightly.
1. 4 Arrange lettuce leaves onto serving plates.
4. Divide the shrimp over the leaves evenly.
5. Garnish with chives and serve immediately.

Shrimp Kabobs

Servings: 3

Preparation Time: 15 minutes

Cooking Time: 8 minutes

Ingredients:

- ¼ cup of olive oil
- 2 tablespoons of fresh lime juice
- ½ chipotle pepper in adobo sauce, seeded and minced
- 1 garlic cloves, minced
- 1½ teaspoon of powdered Erythritol
- ½ teaspoon of red chili powder
- ½ teaspoon of paprika
- ¼ teaspoon of ground cumin
- Salt and ground black pepper, as required
- 1-pound medium raw shrimp, peeled and deveined
- 5 cups of fresh salad greens

Instructions:

1. In a bowl, add all the ingredients except the shrimp and greens and blend well.
2. Add the shrimp and coat with the herb mixture generously.

3. Refrigerate to marinate for at least 30 minutes.
4. Preheat the grill to medium-high heat.
5. Grease the grill grate.
6. Thread the shrimp onto the re-soaked wooden skewers.
7. Place the skewers onto the grill and cook for about 3-4 minutes per side.
8. Remove from the grill and place onto a platter for about 5 minutes before serving.

Shrimp with Zucchini Noodles

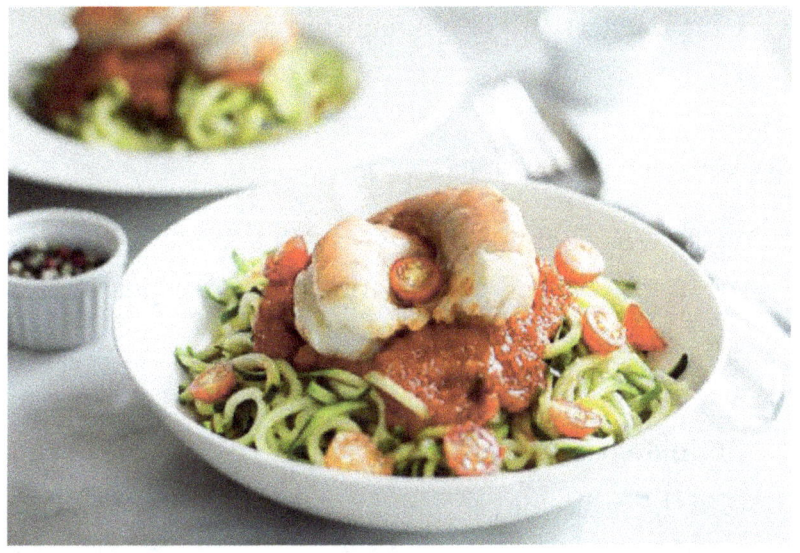

Servings: 4

Preparation Time: 20 minutes

Cooking Time: 8 minutes

Ingredients:

- 2 tablespoons of olive oil
- 1 garlic clove, minced
- ¼ teaspoon of red pepper flakes, crushed
- 1-pound shrimp, peeled and deveined
- Salt and ground black pepper, as required

- 1/3 cup of low-sodium chicken broth
- 2 medium zucchinis, spiralized with a blade
- 1 cup of cherry tomatoes, quartered

Instructions:

1. In a large non-stick skillet, heat the vegetable oil over medium heat and sauté garlic and red pepper flakes for about 1 minute.
2. Add the shrimp, salt and black pepper and cook for about 1 minute per side.
3. Add the broth and zucchini noodles and cook for about 3-4 minutes.
4. Stir in the tomato quarters and take away from the heat.
5. Serve hot.

Shrimp with Spinach

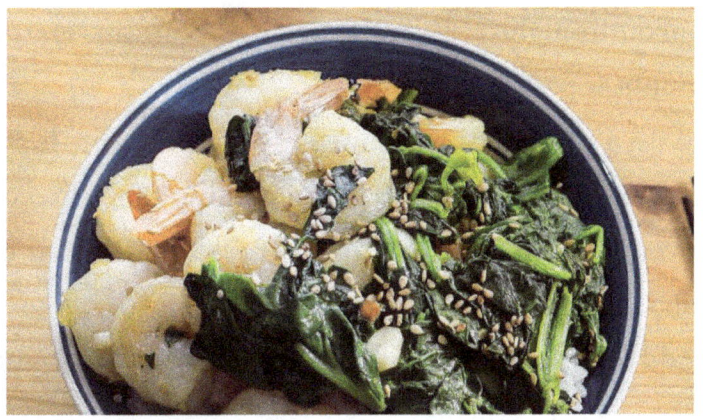

Servings: 4

Preparation Time: 15 minutes

Cooking Time: 9 minutes

Ingredients:

- 3 tablespoons of extra-virgin olive oil
- 1-pound medium shrimp, peeled and deveined
- 1 medium onion, chopped
- 2 garlic cloves, chopped finely
- 1 fresh red chili, sliced
- 1-pound fresh spinach, chopped
- ¼ cup of low-sodium chicken broth

Instructions:

1. In a large non-stick skillet, heat 1 tablespoon of the oil over medium-high heat and cook the shrimp for about 2 minutes per side.
2. With a slotted spoon, transfer the shrimp onto a plate.
3. In the same skillet, heat the remaining 2 tablespoons of oil over medium heat and sauté the garlic and red chili for about 1 minute.
4. Add the spinach and broth and cook for about 2-3 minutes, stirring occasionally.
5. Stir in the cooked shrimp and cook for about 1 minute.
6. Serve hot.

Shrimp with Broccoli & Carrot

Servings: 5

Preparation Time: 15 minutes

Cooking Time: 8 minutes

Ingredients:

For Sauce:

- 1 tablespoon of fresh ginger, grated
- 2 garlic cloves, minced
- 3 tablespoons of low-sodium soy sauce
- 1 tablespoon of balsamic vinegar
- 1 teaspoon of Erythritol
- ¼ teaspoon of red pepper flakes, crushed

For Shrimp Mixture:

- 3 tablespoons of olive oil
- 1½ pounds of medium shrimp, peeled and deveined
- 12 ounces of broccoli florets
- 8 ounces of, carrot, peeled and sliced

Instructions:

1. For sauce: In a bowl, place all the ingredients and beat until well combined. Set aside.
2. In a large wok, heat oil over medium-high heat and cook the shrimp for about 2 minutes, stirring occasionally.
3. Add the broccoli and carrot and cook about 3-4 minutes, stirring frequently.
4. Stir in the sauce mixture and cook for about 1-2 minutes.
5. Serve immediately.

Shrimp, Spinach & Tomato Casserole

Servings: 6

Preparation Time: 15 minutes

Cooking Time: 25 minutes

Ingredients:

- 2 tablespoons of extra-virgin olive oil
- 1 tablespoon of garlic, minced
- 1½ pounds large shrimp, peeled and deveined
- ¾ teaspoon of dried oregano, crushed
- ½ teaspoon of red pepper flakes, crushed
- ¼ cup of fresh spinach, chopped finely
- ¾ cup of low-sodium chicken broth
- 1 tablespoon of fresh lemon juice
- 2 cups of tomatoes, chopped
- 4 ounces of feta cheese, crumbled

Instructions:

1. Preheat your oven to 350 degrees F.
2. In a large skillet, heat the oil over medium-high heat and sauté the garlic for about 1 minute.

3. Add the shrimp, oregano and red pepper flakes and cook for about 4-5 minutes.
4. Stir in the spinach and salt and immediately remove from the heat.
5. Transfer the shrimp mixture into a casserole dish and spread in a good layer.
6. In the same skillet, add the broth and juice over medium heat and simmer for about 3-5 minutes or until reduces to half.
7. Stir in the tomatoes and cook for about 2-3 minutes.
8. Remove from the heat and place the tomato mixture over shrimp mixture evenly.
9. Top with feta cheese evenly.
10. Bake for about 15-20 minutes or until the top becomes golden brown.
11. Serve hot.

Prawns with Bell Pepper

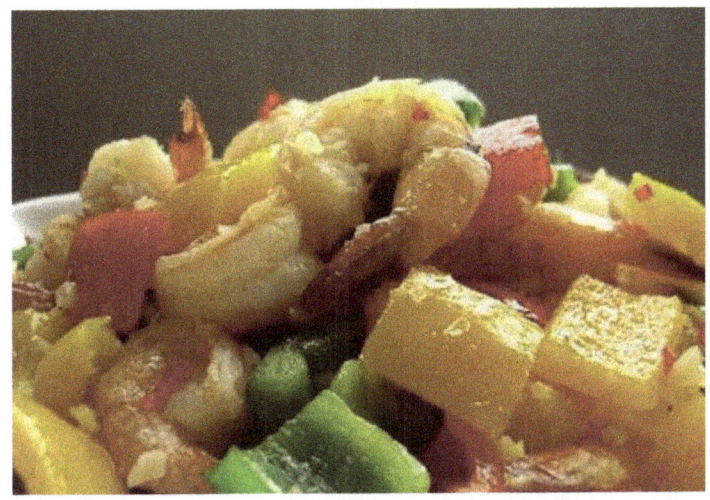

Servings: 4

Preparation Time: 20 minutes

Cooking Time: 8 minutes

Ingredients:

- 2 tablespoons of olive oil
- 4 garlic cloves, minced
- 1 fresh red chili, sliced
- 1-pound prawns, peeled and deveined
- ½ cup of green bell pepper, seeded and julienned
- ½ cup of yellow bell pepper, seeded and julienned

- ½ cup of red bell pepper, seeded and julienned
- ½ cup of orange bell pepper, seeded and julienned
- ½ cup of white onion, sliced thinly
- ¼ cup of low-sodium chicken broth
- Salt and ground black pepper, as required

Instructions:

1. In a large non-stick skillet, heat olive oil over medium heat and sauté the garlic and red chili for about 2 minutes.
2. Add the prawn, bell peppers, onion and black pepper and fry for about 5 minutes.
3. Stir in the broth and cook for about 1 minute.
4. Serve hot.

Prawns with Broccoli

Servings: 4

Preparation Time: 20 minutes

Cooking Time: 10 minutes

Ingredients:

- 2 tablespoons of olive oil, divided
- 1-pound large prawns, peeled and deveined
- ½ of onion, chopped
- 3 garlic cloves, minced
- 3 cups of broccoli floret
- 2 tablespoons of low-sodium soy sauce
- Freshly ground black pepper, as required
- 2 tablespoons of fresh parsley, chopped

Instructions:

1. In a large non-stick skillet, heat 1 tablespoon of olive oil over medium heat and fry the prawns for about 1 minute per side.
2. With a slotted spoon, transfer the prawns onto a plate.

3. In the same skillet, heat the remaining oil over medium heat and sauté the onion and garlic for about 23 minutes.
4. Add the broccoli, soy sauce and black pepper and fry for about 2-3 minutes.
5. Stir in the cooked prawns and fry for about 1-2 minutes.
6. Serve hot.

Prawns with Asparagus

Servings: 4

Preparation Time: 15 minutes

Cooking Time: 13 minutes

Ingredients:

- 3 tablespoons of extra-virgin olive oil
- 1-pound of prawns, peeled and deveined
- 1-pound of asparagus, trimmed
- Salt and ground black pepper, as required
- 1 teaspoon of garlic, minced
- 1 teaspoon of fresh ginger, minced
- 1 tablespoon of low-sodium soy sauce
- 2 tablespoons of lemon juice

Instructions:

1. In a wok, heat 2 tablespoons of oil over medium-high heat and cook the prawns with salt and black pepper for about 3-4 minutes.
2. With a slotted spoon, transfer the prawns into a bowl. Set aside.

3. In the same wok, heat the remaining 1 tablespoon of oil over medium-high heat and cook the asparagus, ginger, garlic, salt and black pepper for about 6-8 minutes, stirring frequently.
4. Stir in the prawns and soy and cook for about 1 minute.
5. Stir in the juice and take away from the heat.
6. Serve hot.

Prawns with Kale

Servings: 4

Preparation Time: 15 minutes

Cooking Time: 20 minutes

Ingredients:

- 1-pound prawns, peeled and deveined
- Salt, as required
- 3 tablespoons of extra-virgin olive oil, divided
- 1 red onion, chopped finely
- 1 fresh red chili, sliced
- 1-pound fresh kale, tough ribs removed and chopped
- 3 tablespoons of low-sodium soy sauce
- 3 tablespoons of fresh orange juice
- 1 tablespoon of orange zest, grated finely
- ½ teaspoon of red pepper flakes, crushed
- Ground black pepper, as required

Instructions:

1. Season the prawns with a little salt.

2. In a large non-stick sauté pan, heat 2 tablespoons of olive oil over high heat and stir-fry the prawns for about 2-3 minutes.
3. With a slotted spoon, transfer the prawns onto a plate.
4. In the same sauté pan, heat the remaining oil over medium heat and sauté the onion for about 4-5 minutes.
5. Add the kale and stir-fry for about 2-3 minutes.
6. With a lid, cover the pan and cook for about 2 minutes.
7. Add the soy sauce, orange juice, zest, red pepper flakes and black pepper and stir to mix well.
8. Stir in the cooked prawns and cook for about 2-3 minutes.
9. Serve hot.

Scallops with Broccoli

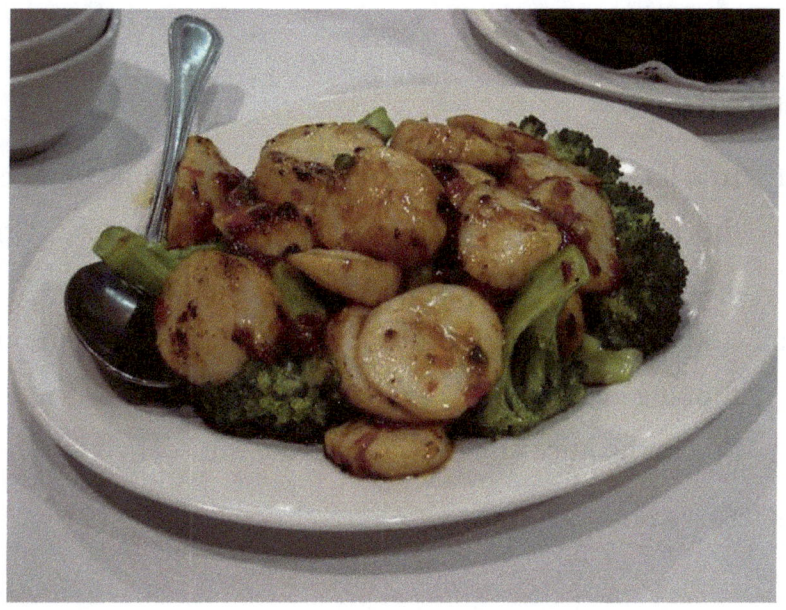

Servings: 2

Preparation Time: 15 minutes

Cooking Time: 9 minutes

Ingredients:

- 2 tablespoons of olive oil
- 1 cup of broccoli, cut into small pieces
- 1 garlic clove, crushed
- ½ pound scallops

- 1 teaspoon of fresh lemon juice
- Salt, as required

Instructions:

1. In a large skillet, heat the oil over medium heat and cook the broccoli and garlic for about 3-4 minutes, stirring occasionally.
2. Add in the scallops and cook for about 3-4 minutes, flipping occasionally.
3. Stir in the juice and take away from the heat.
4. Serve hot.

Scallops with Asparagus

Servings: 5

Preparation Time: 15 minutes

Cooking Time: 10 minutes

Ingredients:

- 2 tablespoons of olive oil
- ¼ cup of yellow onion, chopped
- 2 garlic cloves, minced
- 2 tablespoons of fresh rosemary, minced
- 1-pound fresh asparagus, trimmed and cut into 1-inch pieces
- 2 teaspoons of fresh lemon zest, grated
- 1½ pounds baby scallops
- Salt and ground black pepper, as required
- 2 tablespoons of fresh lemon juice

Instructions:

1. In a large skillet, heat the oil over medium-high heat and sauté the onion for about 2 minutes.
2. Add the garlic and rosemary and sauté for about 1 minute.

3. Add the asparagus and lemon peel and cook for about 1-2 minutes.
4. Add the scallops and stir to mix.
5. Immediately reduce the heat to medium and cook, covered for about 4-5 minutes, stirring occasionally.
6. Stir in lemon juice, salt and black pepper and take away from the heat.
7. Serve hot.

Scallops with Spinach

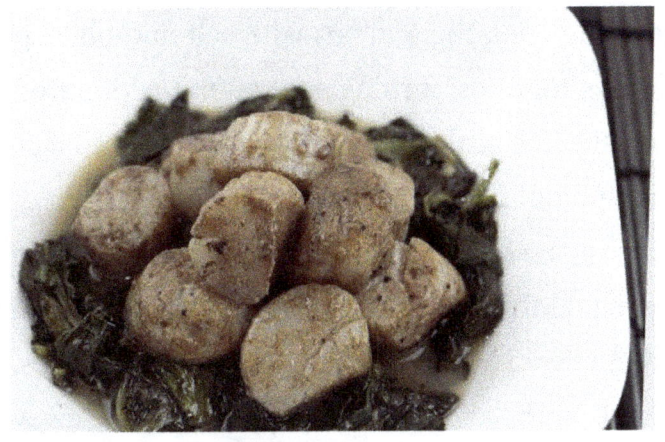

Servings: 5

Preparation Time: 15 minutes

Cooking Time: 21 minutes

Ingredients:

- 1 tablespoon of olive oil
- 1½ pounds jumbo sea scallops
- Salt and ground black pepper, as required
- 1 cup of onion, chopped
- 6 garlic cloves, minced
- 14 ounces of fresh baby spinach

Instructions:

1. In a large non-stick skillet, heat the oil over medium-high heat and cook the scallops with salt and black pepper for about 5 minutes, turning once after 2½ minutes.
2. Transfer the scallops into another bowl and canopy them with a bit of foil to stay warm.
3. In the same skillet, add onion and garlic over medium heat and sauté the onion and garlic for about 3 minutes.
4. Add the spinach and cook for about 2-3 minutes.
5. Season with salt and black pepper and take away from the heat.
6. Divide the spinach onto serving plates.
7. Top with scallops and serve immediately.

Shrimp & Scallops with Veggies

Servings: 5

Preparation Time: 20 minutes

Cooking Time: 11 minutes

Ingredients:

- 3 tablespoons of olive oil, divided
- 1-pound of fresh asparagus, cut into 2-inch pieces
- 2 red bell peppers, seeded and chopped
- ¾ pound of medium raw shrimp, peeled and deveined
- ¾ pound of raw scallops
- 1 tablespoon of dried parsley
- ½ teaspoon of garlic, minced
- Salt and freshly ground black pepper, to taste

Instructions:

1. In a large skillet, heat 1 tablespoon of oil over medium heat and stir-fry the asparagus and bell peppers for about 4-5 minutes.
2. With a slotted spoon, transfer the vegetables onto a plate.

3. In the same skillet, heat the remaining oil over medium heat and stir-fry shrimp and scallops for about 2 minutes.
4. Stir in the parsley, garlic, salt, and black pepper, and cook for about 1 minute.
5. Add in the cooked vegetables and cook for about 2-3 minutes.
6. Serve hot.

Vegetarian Burgers

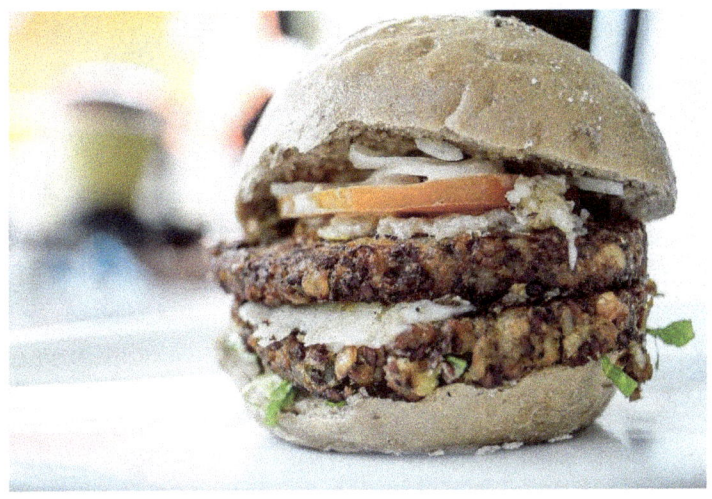

Servings: 4

Preparation Time: 15 minutes

Cooking Time: 16 minutes

Ingredients:

- 1-pound of firm tofu, drained, pressed, and crumbled
- ¾ cup of rolled oats
- ¼ cup of flaxseeds
- 2 cups of frozen spinach, thawed
- 1 medium onion, chopped finely
- 4 garlic cloves, minced

- 1 teaspoon of ground cumin
- 1 teaspoon of red pepper flakes, crushed
- Sea salt and freshly ground black pepper, to taste
- 2 tablespoons of olive oil
- 6 cups of fresh salad greens

Instructions:

1. In a large bowl, add all the ingredients except oil and salad greens and blend until well combined.
2. Put aside for about 10 minutes.
3. Make desired size patties from the mixture.
4. In a nonstick frying pan, heat the oil over medium heat and cook the patties for 6-8 minutes per side.
5. Serve these patties alongside the salad greens.

Cauliflower with Peas

Servings: 4

Preparation Time: 15 minutes

Cooking Time: 15 minutes

Ingredients:

- 2 medium tomatoes, chopped
- ¼ cup of water
- 2 tablespoons of olive oil
- 3 garlic cloves, minced
- ½ tablespoon of fresh ginger, minced
- 1 teaspoon of ground cumin
- 2 teaspoons of ground coriander
- 1 teaspoon of cayenne pepper
- ¼ teaspoon of ground turmeric
- 2 cups of cauliflower, chopped
- 1 cup of fresh green peas, shelled
- Salt and ground black pepper, as required
- ½ cup of warm water

Instructions:

1. In a blender, add tomato and ¼ cup of water and pulse until a smooth puree form. Set aside.
2. In a large skillet, heat the oil over medium heat and sauté the garlic, ginger, green chilies and spices for about 1 minute.
3. Add the cauliflower, peas and tomato puree and cook, stirring for about 3-4 minutes.
4. Add the nice and cosy water and bring to a boil.
5. Reduce the heat to medium-low and cook, covered for about 8-10 minutes or until vegetables are done completely.
6. Serve hot.

Broccoli with Bell Peppers

Servings: 6

Preparation Time: 15 minutes

Cooking Time: 10 minutes

Ingredients:

- 2 tablespoons of olive oil
- 4 garlic cloves, minced
- 1 large white onion, sliced
- 2 cups of small broccoli florets
- 3 red bell peppers, seeded and sliced
- ¼ cup of low-sodium vegetable broth
- Salt and ground black pepper, as required

Instructions:

1. In a large skillet, heat the oil over medium heat and sauté the garlic for about 1 minute.
2. Add the onion, broccoli and bell peppers and fry for about 5 minutes.
3. Add the broth and fry for about 4 minutes more.
4. Serve hot.

Veggies Curry

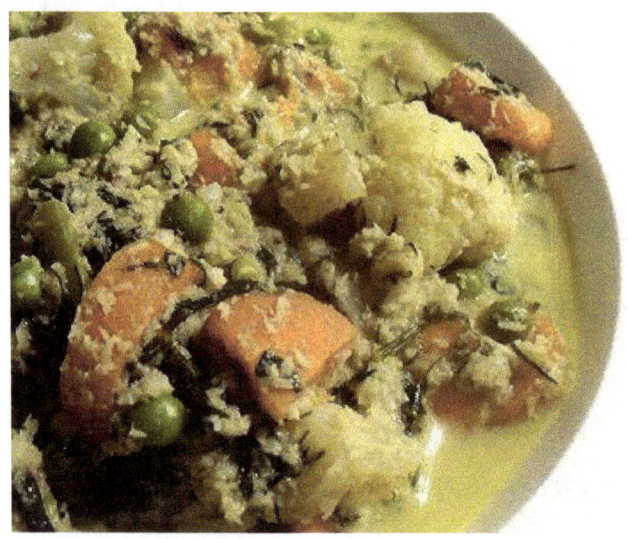

Servings: 6

Preparation Time: 25 minutes

Cooking Time: 15 minutes

Ingredients:

- 1 tablespoon of olive oil
- 1 small yellow onion, chopped
- 1 teaspoon of fresh thyme, chopped
- 1 garlic clove, minced
- 8 ounces of fresh mushroom, sliced
- 1-pound Brussels sprouts

- 3 cups of fresh spinach
- Salt and ground black pepper, as required

Instructions:

1. In a large skillet, heat the oil over medium heat and sauté the onion for about 3-4 minutes.
2. Add the thyme and garlic and sauté for about 1 minute.
3. Add the mushrooms and cook for about 15 minutes or until caramelized.
4. Add the Brussels sprouts and cook for about 2-3 minutes.
5. Stir in the spinach and cook for about 3-4 minutes.
6. Stir in the salt and black pepper and take away from the heat.
7. Serve hot.

Veggies Combo

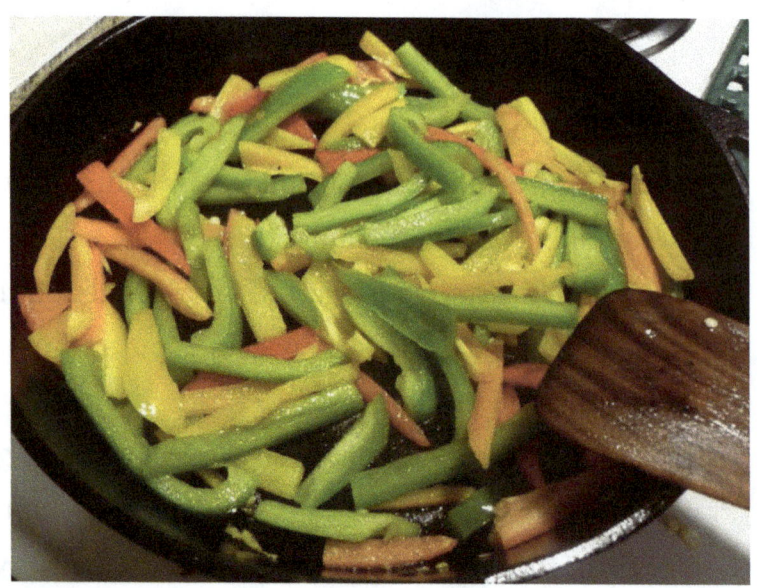

Servings: 4

Preparation Time: 15 minutes

Cooking Time: 10 minutes

Ingredients:

- 1 tablespoon of olive oil
- ½ cup of onion, sliced
- ½ cup of red bell pepper, seeded and julienned
- ½ cup of orange bell pepper, seeded and julienned
- 1½ cups of yellow squash, sliced

- 1½ cups of zucchini, sliced
- 1½ teaspoons of garlic, minced
- ¼ cup of water
- Salt and ground black pepper, as required

Instructions:

1. In a large skillet, heat the oil over medium-high heat and sauté the onion, bell peppers and squash for about 4-5 minutes.
2. Add the garlic and sauté for about 1 minute.
3. Add the remaining ingredients and stir to mix.
4. Reduce the heat to medium and cook for about 3-4 minutes, stirring occasionally.
5. Serve hot.

Cauliflower with Peas

Servings: 4

Preparation Time: 15 minutes

Cooking Time: 15 minutes

Ingredients:

- 2 medium tomatoes, chopped
- ¼ cup of water
- 2 tablespoons of olive oil
- 3 garlic cloves, minced
- ½ tablespoon of fresh ginger, minced
- 1 teaspoon of ground cumin
- 2 teaspoons of ground coriander
- 1 teaspoon of cayenne pepper
- ¼ teaspoon of ground turmeric
- 2 cups of cauliflower, chopped
- 1 cup of fresh green peas, shelled
- Salt and ground black pepper, as required
- ½ cup of warm water

Instructions:

1. In a blender, add tomato and ¼ cup of water and pulse until a smooth puree form. Set aside.
2. In a large wok, heat oil over medium heat and sauté the garlic, ginger, green chilies and spices for about 1 minute.
3. Add the cauliflower, peas and tomato puree and cook, stirring for about 3-4 minutes.
4. Add the nice and cosy water and bring to a boil.
5. Adjust the heat to medium-low and cook, covered for about 8-10 minutes or until vegetables are done completely.
6. Serve hot.

Bok Choy & Mushroom Stir Fry

Servings: 4

Preparation Time: 15 minutes

Cooking Time: 10 minutes

Ingredients:

- 1-pound baby bok choy
- 4 teaspoons of olive oil
- 1 teaspoon of fresh ginger, minced
- 2 garlic cloves, chopped
- 5 ounces of fresh mushrooms, sliced
- 2 tablespoons of red wine
- 2 tablespoons of soy sauce
- Ground black pepper, as required

Instructions:

1. Trim bases of bok choy and separate outer leaves from stalks, leaving the littlest inner leaves attached.
2. In a large cast-iron wok, heat the oil over medium-high heat and sauté the ginger and garlic for about 1 minute.
3. Stir in the mushrooms and cook for about 4-5 minutes, stirring frequently.

4. Stir in the bok choy leaves and stalks and cook for about 1 minute, tossing with tongs.
5. Stir in the wine, soy and black pepper and cook for about 2-3 minutes, tossing occasionally.
6. Serve hot.

Broccoli with Bell Peppers

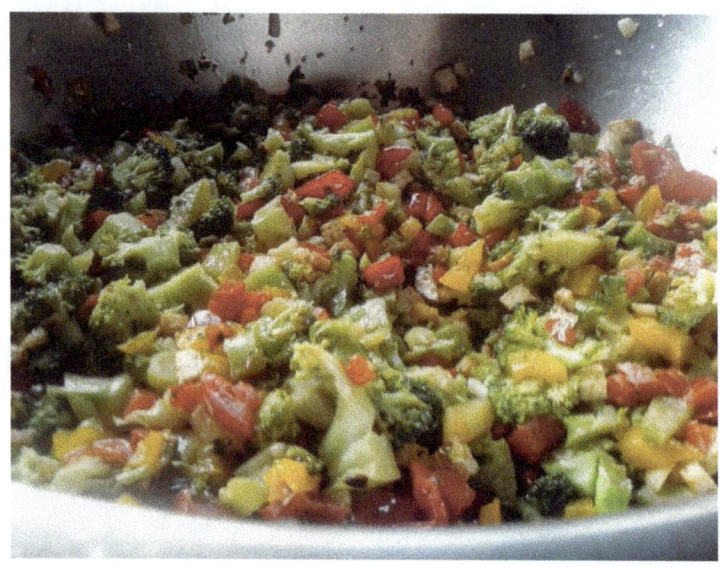

Servings: 6

Preparation Time: 10 minutes

Cooking Time: 10 minutes

Ingredients:

- 2 tablespoons of olive oil
- 4 garlic cloves, minced
- 1 large white onion, sliced
- 2 cups of small broccoli florets
- 3 red bell peppers, seeded and sliced

- ¼ cup of low-sodium vegetable broth
- Salt and ground black pepper, as required

Instructions:

1. In a large wok, heat oil over medium heat and sauté the garlic for about 1 minute.
2. Add the onion, broccoli and bell peppers and cook for about 5 minutes, stirring frequently.
3. Stir in the broth and cook for about 4 minutes, stirring frequently.
4. Stir in the salt and black pepper and take away from the heat.
5. Serve hot.

Stuffed Zucchini

Servings: 8

Preparation Time: 15 minutes

Cooking Time: 18 minutes

Ingredients:

- 4 medium zucchinis, halved lengthwise
- 1 cup of red bell pepper, seeded and minced
- ½ cup of Kalamata olives, pitted and minced
- ½ cup of tomatoes, minced
- 1 teaspoon of garlic, minced
- 1 tablespoon of dried oregano, crushed
- Salt and ground black pepper, as required
- ½ cup of feta cheese, crumbled
- ¼ cup of fresh parsley, chopped finely

Instructions:

1. Preheat your oven to 350 degrees F.
2. Grease a large baking sheet.
3. With a melon baller, scoop out the flesh of every zucchini half. Discard the flesh.

4. In a bowl, mix bell pepper, olives, tomato, garlic, oregano and black pepper.
5. Stuff each zucchini half with the veggie mixture evenly.
6. Arrange zucchini halves onto the prepared baking sheet and Bake for about 15 minutes.
7. Now, set the oven to broiler on high.
8. Top each zucchini half with feta cheese and broil for about 3 minutes.
9. Garnish with parsley and serve hot.

Zucchini & Bell Pepper Curry

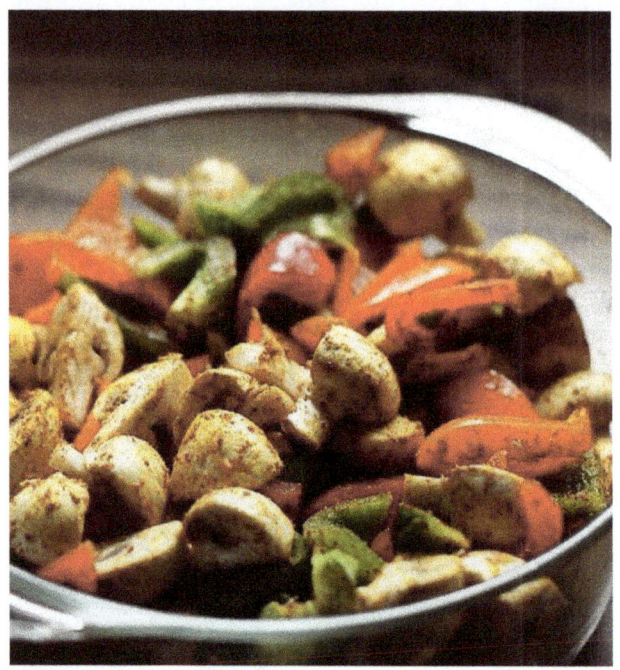

Servings: 6

Preparation Time: 20 minutes

Cooking Time: 20 minutes

Ingredients:

- 2 medium zucchinis, chopped
- 1 green bell pepper, seeded and cubed
- 1 red bell pepper, seeded and cubed

- 1 yellow onion, sliced thinly
- 2 tablespoons of olive oil
- 2 teaspoons of curry powder
- Salt and ground black pepper, as required
- ¼ cup of homemade low-sodium vegetable broth
- ¼ cup of fresh cilantro, chopped

Instructions:

1. Preheat your oven to 375 degrees F.
2. Lightly grease a large baking dish.
3. In a large bowl, add all ingredients except cilantro and blend until well combined.
4. Transfer the vegetable mixture into prepared baking dish.
5. Bake for about 15-20 minutes.
6. Serve immediately with the garnishing of cilantro

Zucchini Noodles with Mushroom Sauce

Servings: 5

Preparation Time: 20 minutes

Cooking Time: 15 minutes

Ingredients:

For Mushroom Sauce:

- 1½ tablespoons of olive oil
- 1 large garlic clove, minced
- 1¼ cups of fresh button mushrooms, sliced
- ¼ cup of homemade low-sodium vegetable broth
- ¼ cup of cream
- Salt and ground black pepper, as to require

For Zucchini Noodles:

- 3 large zucchinis, spiralized with blade C
- ¼ cup of fresh parsley leaves, chopped

Instructions:

1. For mushroom sauce: In a large skillet, heat the oil over medium heat and sauté the garlic for about 1 minute.
2. Stir in the mushrooms and cook for about 6-8 minutes.

3. Stir in the broth and cook for about 2 minutes, stirring continuously.
4. Stir in the cream, salt and black pepper and cook for about 1 minute.
5. Meanwhile, for the zucchini noodles: In a large pan of the boiling water, add the zucchini noodles and cook for about 2-3 minutes.
6. With a slotted spoon, transfer the zucchini noodles into a colander and immediately rinse under cold running water.
7. Drain the zucchini noodles well and transfer onto a large paper towel-lined plate to drain.
8. Divide the zucchini noodles onto serving plates evenly.
9. Remove the sauce from the heat and place over zucchini noodles evenly.
10. Serve immediately with the garnishing of parsley.

Squash Casserole

Servings: 8

Preparation Time: 15 minutes

Cooking Time: 55 minutes

Ingredients:

- ¼ cup of plus
- 2 tablespoons of olive oil, divided
- 1 small yellow onion, chopped
- 3 summer squashes, sliced
- 4 eggs, beaten
- 3 cups of low-fat cheddar cheese, shredded and divided
- 2 tablespoons of unsweetened almond milk
- 2-3 tablespoons of almond flour
- 2 tablespoons of Erythritol
- Salt and ground black pepper, as required

Instructions:

1. Preheat the oven to 375 degrees F.
2. In a large skillet, heat 2 tablespoons of oil over medium heat and cook the onion and squash for about 8-10 minutes, stirring occasionally.

3. Remove the skillet from the heat.
4. Place the eggs, 1 cup of cheddar cheese, almond milk, almond flour, Erythritol, salt and black pepper in a large bowl and blend until well combined.
5. Add the squash mixture, and remaining oil and stir to mix.
6. Transfer the mixture into a large casserole dish and sprinkle with the remaining cheddar cheese.
7. Bake for about 35-45 minutes.
8. Remove the casserole dish from oven and put aside for about 5-10 minutes before serving.
9. Cut into 8 equal-sized portions and serve.

Veggies & Walnut Loaf

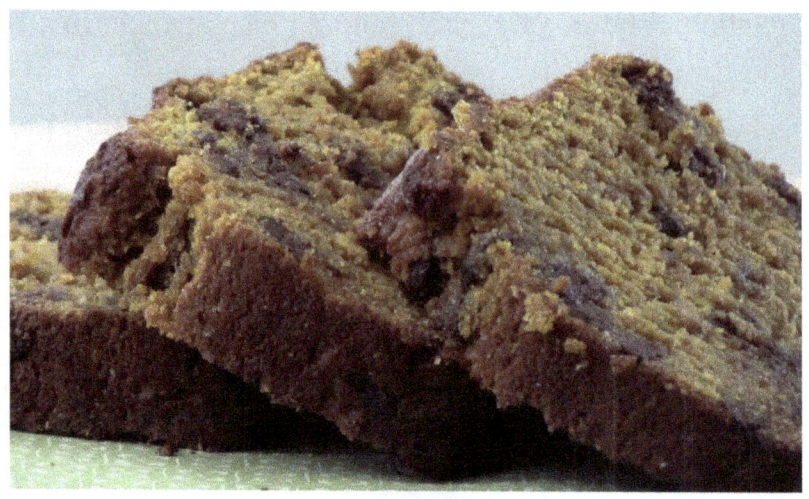

Servings: 10

Preparation Time: 15 minutes

Cooking Time: 1 hour 10 minutes

Ingredients:

- 1 tablespoon of olive oil
- 2 yellow onions, chopped
- 2 garlic cloves, minced
- 1 teaspoon of dried rosemary, crushed
- 1 cup of walnuts, chopped
- 2 large carrots, peeled and chopped

- 1 large celery stalk, chopped
- 1 large green bell pepper, seeded and chopped
- 1 cup of fresh button mushrooms, chopped
- 5 large eggs
- 1¼ cups of almond flour
- Salt and ground black pepper, to taste

Instructions:

1. Preheat your oven to 350-degree F.
2. Line 2 loaf pans with lightly greased parchment papers.
3. In a large wok, heat the vegetable oil over medium heat and sauté the onion for about 4-5 minutes.
4. Add the garlic and rosemary and sauté for about 1 minute.
5. Add the walnuts and vegetables and cook for about 3–4 minutes.
6. Remove the wok from heat and transfer the mixture into a large bowl.
7. Put aside to chill slightly.
8. In another bowl, add the eggs, flour, sea salt, and black pepper, and beat until well combined.
9. Add the egg mixture into the bowl with vegetable mixture and blend until well combined.

10. Divide the mixture into prepared loaf pans evenly.
11. Bake for about 50–60 minutes or until the top becomes golden brown.
12. Remove from the oven and put aside to chill slightly.
13. Carefully invert the loaves onto a platter.
14. Cut into desired sized slices and serve.

Tofu & Veggie Burgers

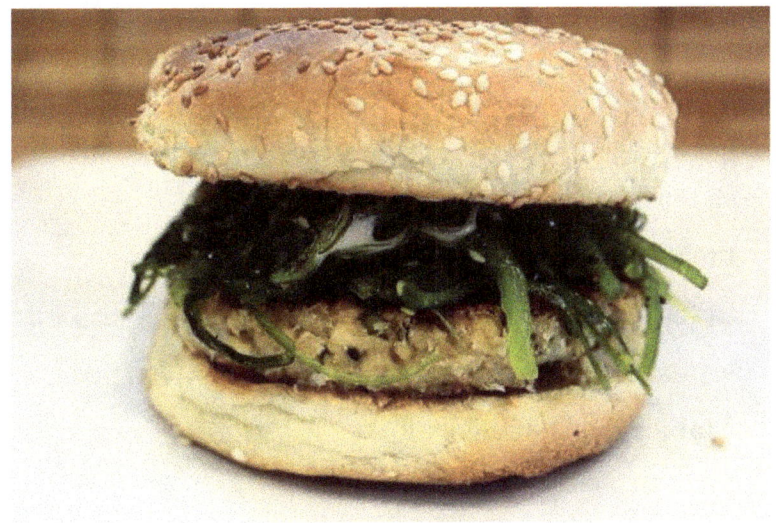

Servings: 2

Preparation Time: 20 minutes

Cooking Time: 8 minutes

Ingredients:

For Patties:

- ½ cup of firm tofu pressed and drained
- 1 medium carrot, peeled and gated
- 1 tablespoon of onion, chopped
- 1 tablespoon of scallion, chopped

- 1 tablespoon of fresh parsley, chopped
- ½ garlic clove, minced
- 2 teaspoons of low-sodium soy sauce
- 1 tablespoon of arrowroot flour
- 1 teaspoon of nutritional yeast flakes
- ½ teaspoon of Dijon mustard
- 1 teaspoon of paprika
- ¼ teaspoon of ground turmeric
- ½ teaspoon of ground black pepper
- 2 tablespoons of olive oil

For Serving:

- ½ cup of cherry tomatoes halved
- 2 cup of fresh baby greens

Instructions:

1. For patties: in a bowl, add the tofu and with a fork, mash well.
2. Add the remaining ingredients apart from oil and blend until well combined.
3. Make 4 equal-sized patties from the mixture.

4. Heat the oil in a frying pan over low heat and cook the patties for about 4 minutes per side.
5. Divide the avocado, tomatoes and greens onto serving plates.
6. Top each plate with 2 patties and serve.

Tofu & Veggie Lettuce Wraps

Servings: 4

Preparation Time: 15 minutes

Cooking Time: 6 minutes

Ingredients:

For Wraps:

- 1 tablespoon of olive oil
- 14 ounces of extra-firm tofu, drained, pressed and cut into cubes
- 1 teaspoon of curry powder
- Salt, as required
- 8 lettuce leaves
- 1 small carrot, peeled and julienned
- ½ cup of radishes, sliced
- 2 tablespoons of fresh cilantro, chopped

For Sauce:

- ½ cup of creamy peanut butter
- 1 tablespoon of maple syrup
- 2 tablespoons of low-sodium soy sauce
- 2 tablespoons of fresh lime juice

- ¼ teaspoon of red pepper flakes, crushed
- ¼ cup of water

Instructions:

1. For tofu: in a skillet, heat the oil over medium heat and cook the tofu, curry powder and a little salt for about 5-6 minutes or until golden brown, stirring frequently.
2. Remove from the heat and put aside to chill slightly.
3. Meanwhile, for sauce: in a bowl, add all the ingredients and beat until smooth.
4. Arrange the lettuce leaves onto serving plates.
5. Divide the tofu, carrot, radish and peanuts over each leaf evenly.
6. Garnish with cilantro and serve alongside the peanut sauce.

Tofu with Kale

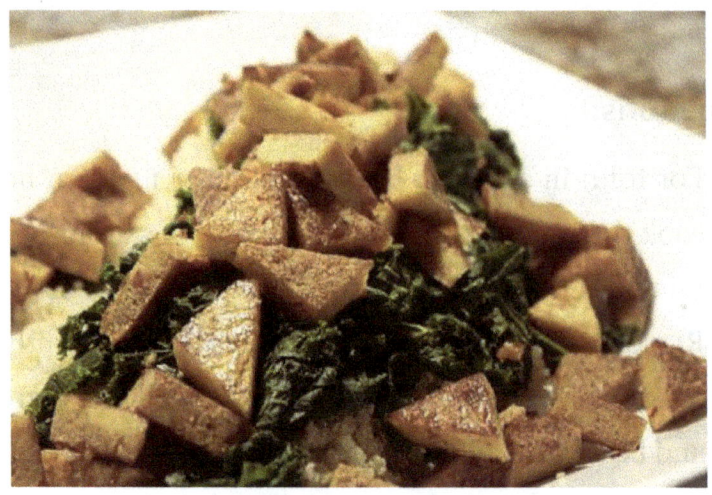

Servings: 2

Preparation Time: 15 minutes

Cooking Time: 10 minutes

Ingredients:

- 1 tablespoon of extra-virgin olive oil
- ½ pound tofu, pressed, drained and cubed
- 1 teaspoon of fresh ginger, minced
- 1 garlic clove, minced
- ¼ teaspoon of red pepper flakes, crushed

- 6 ounces of fresh kale, tough ribs removed and chopped finely
- 1 tablespoon of low-sodium soy sauce

Instructions:

1. In a large non-stick wok, heat vegetable oil over medium-high heat and stir-fry the tofu for about 3-3 minutes.
2. Add the ginger, garlic and red pepper flakes and cook for about 1 minute, stirring continuously.
3. Stir in the kale and soy and stir-fry for about 4-5 minutes.
4. Serve hot.

www.ingramcontent.com/pod-product-compliance
Lightning Source LLC
Chambersburg PA
CBHW070734030426
42336CB00013B/1968